MORNING WORKOUTS FOR WOMEN

Step by Step Fitness Exercise for beginners to Strengthen core, Achieve good Posture, Enhance Flexibility and Maintain balance with less time

Barbara L. Buffington

TABLE OF CONTENT

INTRODUCTION

Kendra was a young woman living in a lively metropolis. Kendra worked long hours at a top law company. Her days were filled with numerous meetings, paperwork, and tight deadlines, leaving her with little time to herself.

Kendra's health deteriorated gradually throughout the months. Every morning, she'd wake up sluggish and exhausted, with her entire body suffering from top to bottom. Even the most basic duties seemed like a nuisance, and she struggled to keep up with her tight schedule.

At first, Kendra dismissed these symptoms as the effects of stress and a lack of sleep. However, as time passed, the pain and weariness appeared to intensify. She developed chronic joint pain, making it impossible for her to walk without agony.

Kendra, concerned about her worsening health, went to consult a doctor. Following a battery of tests and exams, she was diagnosed with a variety of health conditions, many of which were caused by her sedentary lifestyle and lack of exercise.

The doctor said that extended sitting, along with a lack of physical exercise, had taken its toll on her body, resulting in muscular stiffness, weariness, and joint discomfort.

Determined to improve her health, Kendra set out on a mission to discover a remedy. She browsed bookstores and internet forums, looking for strategies to enhance her health.

One day, while wandering at a bookshop, she came upon a book called Morning Workouts for Women.
Kendra was intrigued by the title and decided to acquire the book and read its contents. To her amazement, the book was full of useful information and practical advice on how to live a better lifestyle. It discussed the significance of regular exercise, an adequate diet, and the advantages of remaining active.

Kendra began adopting the book's instructions into her daily routine, eager to put the hidden secrets contained inside its pages into action.

She started by incorporating little exercise sessions into her day, pausing to stretch and move her body. She also changed her diet, choosing healthier meal alternatives and cutting out on processed goods.

Kendra gradually noticed a significant improvement in her health and well-being. The overall body soreness and exhaustion began to fade, replaced by renewed energy and vigor. Her joint pain became more bearable, allowing her to move freely and comfortably.

Kendra was able to regain her health and fitness thanks to the book's advice and her drive to make great changes. Her path served as a reminder that with the correct education and determination, anybody can overcome the limitations of sedentary living and thrive in body, mind, and spirit.

Chapter 1: Understanding the Benefits of Morning Exercise

Morning exercise has various benefits for women, including improved physical, mental, and emotional well-being.

A consistent morning fitness regimen may improve many elements of a woman's life, increasing overall health and vigor. Here's a complete look at the benefits of morning exercise for women.

Increased Energy Levels: Physical exercise in the morning jumpstarts the body's metabolism, resulting in more energy throughout the day.

Women who exercise in the morning frequently report feeling more awake, focused, and prepared to face everyday challenges.

Improved Mood: Research has revealed that morning exercise causes the production of endorphins, neurotransmitters important for emotions of happiness and well-being. Women who exercise in the morning are more likely to have a better mood and less stress throughout the day.

Regular morning workouts can help with weight control by increasing metabolism and encouraging fat burning. Women who exercise in the morning may have an easier time maintaining a healthy weight and meeting their fitness objectives.

Better Mental Clarity: Morning exercise provides cognitive advantages, such as increased mental clarity and attention. Women who begin their days with physical activity frequently report feeling more intellectually aware and productive throughout the day.

Increased Strength and Endurance: Consistent morning exercise can help you gain strength, endurance, and general fitness. Women who emphasize early workouts may see improvements in muscular tone and athletic performance over time.

Exercise can help women maintain hormonal balance, which is critical for general health and well-being. Morning exercise can help stabilize hormone levels, resulting in better mood, energy, and general hormonal health.

Better Sleep Quality: Morning exercise can improve sleep quality by regulating the body's natural sleep-wake cycle. Women who exercise in the morning often have deeper, more peaceful sleep, which leads to better overall health and energy.

Morning exercise has several benefits for women, including greater energy, improved mood, improved weight management, higher mental clarity, increased strength and endurance, controlled hormonal balance, and better sleep quality.

Women who incorporate regular morning workouts into their routines can improve their physical, mental, and emotional well-being, resulting in a better and more rewarding existence.

Overcoming Common Challenges and Excuses

Morning exercises for women have various benefits, including greater energy, improved mood, and productivity throughout the day. However, many women struggle to stick to a steady morning workout practice owing to a variety of barriers and reasons.

By tackling these frequent problems head on and applying practical techniques, women may overcome them and get the advantages of early exercise.

1. Lack of Motivation: Getting out of bed early to exercise can be challenging, especially when conflicting demands and duties are present.

To overcome this difficulty, create precise, attainable objectives and remind yourself of the benefits of early exercise, such as greater energy and improved mood.

2. *Time constraints:* Juggling job, family, and other responsibilities often leave little time for exercise. To make morning exercises more realistic, consider waking up somewhat earlier or including quick and efficient workouts that can be done in a short period of time, such as high-intensity interval training (HIIT) or circuit training.

3. *Fatigue:* Waking up fatigued might reduce motivation and make it difficult to exercise. To counteract weariness, emphasize quality sleep by sticking to a predictable sleep schedule and developing a pleasant nighttime ritual. Start your morning with a good meal and drink plenty of water to enhance your energy levels.

4. *Weather Conditions:* Bad weather, such as rain or freezing temperatures, might discourage women from exercising outside. In such instances, prepare an alternative plan for indoor workouts, such as watching an internet fitness video or participating in indoor hobbies like yoga or dancing.

5. *Lack of responsibility:* Without external responsibility, it's easy to find excuses and miss morning workouts. To keep accountable, find a workout companion or enroll in a fitness program with planned sessions. Alternatively, track your progress and celebrate your accomplishments to keep motivated.

6. *Perfectionism:* Feeling the need to have a flawless exercise or stick to a rigorous program can add unneeded stress and contribute to procrastination. Instead, strive for consistency rather than perfection, and be adaptable with your workout regimen to accommodate changes in schedule or preferences.

By tackling these typical hurdles and excuses, women may overcome obstacles to morning exercises and get the physical and emotional advantages of regular exercise, laying the groundwork for a productive and joyful day ahead.

Setting Goals and Establishing a Morning Routine

Setting objectives and creating a daily routine are critical for personal development and productivity. This is especially true for women, who typically have many duties.

Women who begin their day with a well-planned routine can set the tone for a good day ahead. Morning workouts are an important part of this schedule.

Setting defined goals is critical. Whether it's increasing fitness, lowering weight, or boosting general well-being, well-stated goals give guidance and incentive.

Goals should be SMART (specific, measurable, achievable, relevant, and time-bound). For example, a goal may be to do a 30-minute workout every morning for the next month.

Second, creating a morning fitness regimen that is personalized to individual preferences and schedules is critical. This regimen should include a variety of aerobic activities, weight training, flexibility exercises, and mindfulness techniques.

Cardiovascular workouts such as vigorous walking, running, or cycling increase heart rate and endurance. Strength training with bodyweight movements or low weights improves muscular tone and metabolism. Flexibility exercises like yoga or stretching routines enhance mobility and lower the chance of injury.

Adding mindfulness activities like meditation or deep breathing exercises improves brain clarity and decreases stress.

Third, developing a regular morning routine is critical to long-term success. This entails rising up at a same time every day, preferably early enough to fit in a complete training session before other obligations arise. Creating a supportive atmosphere by laying out training clothing the night before, cooking a good meal, and setting up a specific workout area all help with adherence to the practice.

Tracking progress is critical for remaining accountable and inspired. Keeping a workout diary or using fitness apps to document exercises, measure progress, and celebrate accomplishments increases motivation and gives useful feedback.

Setting objectives and creating a full morning routine, including workouts adapted to individual requirements, is critical for women seeking to live healthy, balanced lives. Consistency, adaptation, and self-awareness are essential qualities in this road to personal well-being and success.

Chapter 2: The Importance of Warm-Up and Mobility

Starting your day with exercise may set a positive tone for the remainder of the day, especially for women who want to stay healthy and active. However, before beginning any training plan, emphasize warm-up and mobility activities to properly prepare your body.

1. *Injury Prevention:* Women, like everyone else, are prone to injuries during exercises, especially if their bodies are not well prepared.

Warming up boosts blood flow to the muscles, making them more supple and less susceptible to strains or rips. Mobility exercises that focus on joint motions improve flexibility and lower the risk of injury due to the limited range of motion.

2. *Improved Performance:* A complete warm-up prepares your body for peak performance throughout exercise. It progressively increases heart rate, improving circulation and oxygen supply to muscles.

This trains muscles to operate more efficiently, resulting in increased strength, endurance, and overall performance. Mobility exercises keep joints moving smoothly, allowing for good form and increasing training efficacy.

3. *Mental Preparation:* Morning exercises can be difficult, especially when starting the day on a tight schedule. Warm-up activities help as a transition from rest to action, psychologically preparing ladies for the next workout.

It improves attention, decreases tension, and promotes mood, establishing a pleasant attitude for the day.

4. *Long-Term Benefits:* Including warm-up and mobility exercises in morning routines on a regular basis can have a long-term positive impact on women's health.

Improved flexibility and mobility minimize the incidence of age-related joint disorders while also improving total functional fitness, resulting in a healthier and more active lifestyle as individuals age.

Warm-up and mobility exercises in women's morning workouts are critical for injury prevention, improved performance, mental preparation, and long-term health advantages.

Women who devote time to properly preparing their bodies can increase the efficiency of their exercises and lay the groundwork for a healthy lifestyle.

Dynamic Stretching for Flexibility and Joint Health

Dynamic stretching is an essential part of any workout program, particularly for women wanting to improve flexibility and joint health.

Unlike static stretching, which requires retaining a stretch for a lengthy period of time, dynamic stretching uses continuous movement to stretch muscles and enhance range of motion.

Incorporating dynamic stretching into morning exercises can help to establish a good tone for the day by preparing the body for activities and supporting overall health.

Dynamic stretching works numerous muscle groups at once, making it an effective approach to preparing the body for activity. It entails motions that imitate those of the activity to be performed, enhancing muscular flexibility and lowering the chance of injury. For women who often juggle many obligations throughout the day, beginning the day with dynamic stretching can boost energy and improve attention.

Women's dynamic stretching routines may include activities like arm circles, leg swings, hip circles, and torso twists. These motions work both the upper and lower bodies, increasing flexibility in crucial regions such as the shoulders, hips, and spine.

Including dynamic stretches that focus on balance and stability can help women gain core strength, improve posture, and reduce their chance of falling while going about their everyday activities.

In terms of joint health, dynamic stretching lubricates the joints by boosting synovial fluid production, reducing friction and allowing for smoother mobility. This is especially advantageous for women, who are more susceptible to illnesses such as osteoarthritis, which can impair joint mobility and general quality of life.

Women who incorporate dynamic stretching into their daily practice can proactively improve joint health and reduce the impact of age-related changes.

Overall, dynamic stretching is an effective strategy for women looking to improve flexibility and joint health.

Women who incorporate these exercises into their morning routines can benefit from increased range of motion, lower injury risk, and better general well-being throughout the day.

Mobility Exercises to Enhance Range of Motion

Improving your range of motion is critical for general flexibility, joint health, and injury avoidance. Incorporating targeted mobility exercises into your morning routine may greatly enhance your daily movement patterns and general well-being, especially for women who must balance several duties and prioritize their physical health.

Neck Rotations: Move your neck in a circular manner, first clockwise, then counterclockwise. Perform 8–10 rotations on each side to relieve tension and enhance neck mobility, which is necessary for good posture throughout the day.

To do shoulder circles, stand erect and rotate your shoulders forward in a circular motion for 8-10 times before reversing direction. This exercise helps to stretch stiff shoulder muscles and promote flexibility, which is especially good for women who work long hours at desks or carry children.

Spinal Twists: Sit on the edge of a chair, feet flat on the floor. Place your right hand against the back of the chair and your left hand on your right knee.

Gently rotate your body to the right and glance over your right shoulder.Switch sides after holding for 15-20 seconds. This exercise increases spinal mobility and lowers back stress.

To do hip circles, stand with feet hip-width apart and hands on hips. Circle your hips clockwise for 8-10 reps, then counterclockwise. Hip circles enhance hip flexibility and mobility, which are necessary for many daily movements such as walking, squatting, and bending.

Ankle Circles: Sit on the floor with legs outstretched. Point your toes and spin your ankles in a circular manner, starting clockwise and ending counterclockwise. Perform 8-10 rotations each way to enhance ankle mobility, which is essential for maintaining balance and stability.

Incorporating these mobility exercises into your morning routine will not only improve your range of motion, but will also establish a good tone for the day ahead, ensuring that you begin the day feeling limber, motivated, and ready to face whatever difficulties may arise.

To enhance the effectiveness of each exercise, remember to do it with control and good form.

Foam Rolling and Self-Myofascial Release Techniques

Foam rolling and self-myofascial release techniques have become essential components of women's morning exercises for increasing flexibility, reducing muscular tightness, and improving overall performance.

Incorporating these techniques into your daily routine can give you several advantages, both immediate and long-term.

Foam rolling is a technique that uses a cylindrical foam roller to apply pressure to particular muscle regions, focusing on stiffness or pain.

This method reduces tension in the fascia, the connective tissue that surrounds muscles, allowing for more flexibility and range of motion. Self-myofascial release techniques, such as employing massage or lacrosse balls, provide a more specific approach to addressing knots and trigger points in muscle tissue.

Including foam rolling and self-myofascial release in your morning workout routine can help prepare your body for activity by boosting blood flow to the muscles, improving flexibility and lowering the chance of injury during future activities.

These strategies help reduce muscular pain and stiffness, making it simpler to move and complete exercises in perfect form.

To successfully combine foam rolling and self-myofascial release into your morning exercises, begin with a quick warm-up to stimulate blood flow to the muscles.

Then, for 5-10 minutes, target key muscular groups such the calves, quadriceps, hamstrings, glutes, and back.

Roll each muscle group gently and methodically, pausing to apply light pressure to any sore or tight regions until the tension is released.

After your workout, spend an extra 5-10 minutes foam rolling and self-myofascial release to assist minimize muscle discomfort and enhance healing.

Concentrate on regions that seem especially tight or overworked throughout your workout, adjusting the pressure as needed to obtain a pleasant yet effective stretch.

Including foam rolling and self-myofascial release methods into your morning training regimen will aid with flexibility, muscular pain, and overall performance.

By devoting only a few minutes every day to these routines, you may reap tremendous advantages that help you achieve your overall health and fitness objectives.

Chapter 3: Cardiovascular Health and Endurance Training

Cardiovascular health is critical for general well-being, particularly among women. Endurance exercise is essential for strengthening cardiovascular health, and early workouts provide various advantages.

Let's look at the specifics of cardiovascular health, endurance training, and the benefits of early exercise for women.

Cardiovascular Health:

Women are predisposed to a variety of cardiovascular disorders, making it critical to prioritize heart health. Cardiovascular disorders, including heart attacks and strokes, are the leading causes of death among women globally.

Age, family history, lifestyle choices, and hormone variations all have an influence on a woman's cardiovascular health.

Endurance Training:

Endurance training aims to improve cardiovascular fitness and stamina via prolonged physical exercise. It includes activities such as running, cycling, swimming, and aerobic exercise.

Endurance exercise increases heart function, circulation, blood pressure regulation, and overall cardiovascular efficiency. Regular endurance exercise also helps with weight control, decreases stress, and improves mental health.

Morning Workouts For Women:

Morning workouts have special benefits for women who want to improve their cardiovascular health through endurance training. For starters, exercising in the morning boosts metabolism, which helps with weight management and fat reduction.

Second, early workouts increase energy levels, establishing a good tone for the day ahead. Third, morning exercise improves mental clarity and productivity, which benefits general well-being.

Furthermore, morning exercises integrate perfectly into women's everyday routines, promoting consistency and commitment to training plans. Furthermore, exercising in the morning gives you a sense of achievement, which sets a good mood for the rest of the day.

Women should prioritize their cardiovascular health through endurance exercise. Morning exercises are a handy and efficient method to include endurance training into everyday routines, with various advantages to general health and well-being.

Embracing early exercises can help women achieve optimal cardiovascular health and fitness.

Low-Impact Cardio Options for Joint Health

Morning exercises are a great way for ladies to start their day off with energy and vibrancy. For people with joint issues, low-impact aerobic workouts provide a safe and effective fitness regimen.

These exercises are easy on the joints while still giving a heart-pounding workout. Here are some extensive and detailed low-impact cardio solutions designed for women's joint health:

Walking: Begin your day with a quick walk, whether outside or on a treadmill. Walking is a low-impact activity that boosts cardiovascular health and improves lower-body muscles without placing too much strain on the joints.

Cycling is a fantastic low-impact cardio choice, whether done inside or outdoors. It increases leg strength, promotes heart health, and is easy on the knees and hips.

Swimming: Dive into a pool for a relaxing swim. Swimming is a full-body exercise that works many muscle groups while putting minimal strain on the joints. It's especially helpful for women who have arthritis or joint discomfort.

Elliptical Training: Using an elliptical machine gives you a low-impact cardio workout that simulates the motion of walking or jogging without disturbing your joints. It emphasizes the legs, glutes, and arms while protecting the joints.

Rowing machines provide a whole body exercise that builds muscles, increases cardiovascular endurance, and improves joint flexibility. Rowing's smooth, fluid action reduces pressure on the joints, making it an excellent choice for ladies with joint concerns.

Yoga: Including yoga in your morning practice helps enhance joint flexibility, balance, and general health. Gentle yoga postures and sequences stretch and develop muscles without stressing the joints.

Tai Chi: This ancient Chinese martial art focuses on gentle, flowing motions that improve balance, flexibility, and joint health. Tai Chi is appropriate for women of all ages and fitness levels, making it a great low-impact cardiovascular exercise for joint health.

Incorporating these low-impact aerobic activities into your daily routine will help women maintain joint health while also reaping the advantages of regular exercise. Remember to listen to your body, start carefully, and gradually increase the intensity to avoid overexertion and maintain a consistent training regimen.

Interval Training for Increased Stamina

Interval training is a highly efficient way to increase stamina, especially for women who work out in the morning. This method mixes high-intensity bursts of activity with intervals of rest or low-intensity exercise.

It is comprehensive, focusing on numerous fitness components such as cardiovascular endurance, muscular strength, and even mental resilience.

Morning workouts have various advantages for women, such as greater energy throughout the day, higher metabolism, and improved mood. Incorporating interval training into these early routines can increase the advantages.

The intensity of interval training tests the cardiovascular system, resulting in enhanced heart health and stamina over time.

To begin, warm up with dynamic stretches that prepare the muscles and joints for movement.

Then, alternate between short bursts of high-intensity activity, such as sprinting, jumping jacks, or burpees, and brief recovery periods of low-intensity activities, such as walking or running.

This cycle can be performed several times, progressively increasing the intensity or duration of the high-intensity periods as stamina develops.

Interval training is time-saving, making it ideal for hectic mornings. A 20-30-minute workout can provide considerable advantages, including increased cardiovascular capacity and endurance. Furthermore, the afterburn effect, in which the body continues to burn calories at a higher rate after an exercise, helps with weight control objectives.

Interval training provides women with a varied choice of workouts that can be adapted to their fitness levels and goals. Whether it's indoor cycling, bodyweight circuits, or HIIT courses, you can tailor your workout to your specific needs and timetable.

Interval training requires consistent effort to obtain its benefits. Women who incorporate it into their morning routines may progressively build stamina, increase energy levels, and improve general fitness, setting a positive tone for the day ahead.

Furthermore, correct hydration and nutrition are vital for performance and recuperation, guaranteeing long-term success in stamina development.

Outdoor Activities: Walking, Hiking, and Cycling

Outdoor activities such as walking, hiking, and cycling provide a variety of advantages for both physical and mental health. These activities not only raise heart rates but also allow you to immerse yourself in nature's grandeur while instilling a spirit of adventure and discovery.

A brisk morning stroll is a low-impact activity for women of all fitness levels. It helps with weight loss, strengthens bones and muscles, and enhances heart health.

Walking also improves mood and lowers stress, making it an excellent alternative for individuals looking for a relaxing start to the day. Whether it's a relaxing stroll through a neighborhood park or a strenuous walk along gorgeous trails, the possibilities are unlimited.

Hiking is a great option for ladies looking for a difficult workout that also allows them to appreciate beautiful natural settings. Hiking paths provide a variety of terrain to encounter, ranging from undulating hills to steep mountains.

This action not only improves strength and endurance, but it also promotes mental clarity and a sense of success when one achieves new heights. Proper equipment and hydration are vital for a safe and pleasurable hiking trip.

Cycling is a dynamic exercise that provides a full-body workout without straining the joints. Women can select between road cycling for speed and endurance and mountain biking for an exhilarating off-road experience. Cycling boosts cardiovascular fitness, leg strength, and coordination while also increasing mental awareness and reducing stress. Morning riding rides with the wind in their hair and the countryside zipping by are sure to stimulate and inspire.

Including outdoor activities such as walking, hiking, and cycling in morning routines can dramatically improve women's overall health and wellness.shoes

 Whether you're looking for peace and quiet, adventure, or a combination of the two, these activities give a welcome reprieve from indoor routines while also encouraging a deeper connection with nature.

So, lace up your , take a water bottle, and get outside to enjoy the beauty and advantages of the great outdoors.

Chapter 4: Strength Training for Bone Health and Muscle Tone

Strength training is an essential component of a well-rounded fitness routine, with several advantages for bone health and muscle tone, particularly for women. Morning exercises are a great way to start the day with energy and focus.

Here's a detailed guide to understanding the benefits of strength training for bone health and muscle tone, as well as suggestions for successful morning exercises for women.

Strength training, or resistance exercise, strengthens and densifies bones. This is especially important for women, as they are more susceptible to osteoporosis, a disorder characterized by weaker bones. Women who engage in regular strength training can increase bone density and lower their risk of fractures and osteoporosis later in life.

Strength training improves both bone strength and muscle tone, resulting in a more defined body. Contrary to widespread opinion, women will not gain muscle mass from weightlifting unless they train specifically for hypertrophy.

Instead, they'll have a sculpted appearance with more muscular definition. Furthermore, increased muscle mass stimulates metabolism, which aids in weight control and improves overall physical performance.

Morning exercises for women have various benefits, including enhanced metabolism, improved mood and productivity, and better adherence to an exercise plan. To get the most out of early strength training sessions:

Prepare the night before: Lay out your exercise clothing, set up your equipment, and have pre-workout food available.

Warm up your muscles and joints by performing dynamic stretches or a quick aerobic workout.

For optimal efficiency, focus on compound movements such as squats, lunges, push-ups, and deadlifts.

improvement progressively: Begin with lesser weights and progressively increase resistance as strength increases to minimize injury and assure continuous improvement.

Stay Hydrated: Drink water before, during, and after your workout to stay hydrated and perform optimally.

Women who incorporate strength training into their morning exercises may improve bone health, shape their muscles, and set a good tone for the day ahead. With consistency and perseverance, the advantages of strength training will become apparent, resulting in better overall health and wellness.

Resistance Exercises for Building Strength Safely

Morning workouts for women are an excellent way to kick out the day with energy and vibrancy. Incorporating resistance workouts into your morning regimen will help you gain strength, boost metabolism, and enhance overall health.

Here's a thorough guide to resistance workouts designed specifically for women to safely gain strength.

Bodyweight Squats: Begin with your feet hip-width apart and lower into a squat position by bending your knees and pulling your hips back. Maintain a raised chest and balance your weight on your heels. Aim for three sets of 10–15 repetitions.

Push-Ups: Start in a plank posture, hands slightly wider than shoulder width apart. Lower your body until your chest is almost touching the floor, then push back up to the starting position. If necessary, perform knee push-ups as an alternative. Aim for three sets of 8 to 12 repetitions.

Dumbbell Lunges: With a dumbbell in each hand, take a step forward with one leg and lower your body until both knees are bent at 90 degrees.

Push back up to the starting position, then repeat with the other leg. Aim for three sets of ten to twelve repetitions each leg.

Plank: Begin in a forearm plank posture, maintaining your body straight from head to heels. Hold for 30–60 seconds, concentrating on activating your core muscles and keeping appropriate posture.

Dumbbell Rows: Hold a dumbbell in each hand and tilt forward at the hips, keeping your knees slightly bent. Pull the dumbbells up to your chest while pulling your shoulder blades together at the peak of the exercise. Aim for three sets of ten to twelve repetitions each arm.

Deadlifts: Place your feet hip-width apart and grasp a dumbbell or kettlebell in each hand in front of your thighs.

Hinge at the hips while maintaining your back flat, and descend the weights to the ground. To return to a standing position, drive through your heels. Aim for three sets of 8 to 10 repetitions.

Targeting Key Muscle Groups for Functional Fitness

When it comes to morning workouts for women, focusing on major muscle groups for functional fitness is critical for overall health and strength.

Functional fitness focuses on exercises that mirror everyday tasks, hence increasing balance, flexibility, and strength in real-life settings. Incorporating workouts that target certain muscle groups results in a well-rounded fitness plan.

Lower Body: Begin with squats, lunges, and deadlifts to work the glutes, quadriceps, hamstrings, and calves. These motions increase lower body strength, stability, and mobility, which are essential for tasks such as walking, climbing stairs, and carrying groceries.

Planks, Russian twists, and bicycle crunches all help to engage the core muscles. A strong core improves posture, spine support, and balance, making it easier to lift items and stay stable throughout daily motions.

Upper Body: Use push-ups, rows, and shoulder presses to build your chest, back, shoulders, and arms. This increases upper-body strength and endurance, making it easier to handle children, carry bags, and reach above.

Improve balance and stability by including workouts such as single-leg deadlifts, stability ball exercises, and yoga postures such as tree pose. Improved balance lowers the chance of falls and injuries while increasing confidence and ease in daily activities.

Flexibility: Use dynamic stretches and yoga poses to improve flexibility in main muscle groups. Improved flexibility helps to maintain a complete range of motion, reducing stiffness and pain during daily motions.

Cardiovascular Health: Cardiovascular workouts such as brisk walking, running, or cycling can help enhance heart health and endurance. A strong cardiovascular system improves overall fitness and provides more energy throughout the day.

Morning workouts for women enhance functional fitness by targeting important muscle groups with a variety of exercises, improving strength, flexibility, balance, and cardiovascular health for peak performance in everyday activities.

Incorporating these exercises into your morning routine sets a positive tone for the day, increasing energy and general well-being.

Bodyweight Exercises for Functional Strength

Bodyweight exercises are an effective and accessible technique to increase functional strength, making them excellent for women's morning workouts.

These workouts use your own body weight as resistance and require minimal equipment and space. Here's a thorough list of bodyweight exercises for functional strength:

Squats: Begin with your feet shoulder-width apart, then lower your body as if sitting back in a chair, keeping your chest up and your knees behind your toes.

Squats work your quadriceps, hamstrings, and glutes, increasing lower body strength required for daily actions such as lifting and bending.

Push-Ups: Start in a plank posture with your hands shoulder-width apart, then lower your body until your chest almost touches the ground before pushing back up. Push-ups work the chest, shoulders, and triceps, increasing upper-body strength and stability.

Lunges: Stand with your feet together, take one step forward, then lower your body until both knees are bent at a 90-degree angle before returning to the starting position. Lunges work the quadriceps, hamstrings, and glutes, enhancing balance and coordination.

Planks: Begin in a push-up position, elbows bent and resting on the forearms, and maintain a straight line from head to heels. Planks work the core muscles, particularly the abs and obliques, which improves stability and posture.

Glute Bridges: Lie on your back with knees bent and feet flat on the ground, lift your hips to the ceiling while clenching your glutes, and then drop back down. Glute bridges strengthen the glutes and lower back, increasing hip stability and decreasing the incidence of lower back injury.

Incorporate these exercises into women's morning routines to improve functional strength, metabolism, and energy levels throughout the day. Aim for three sets of 10-15 repetitions for each exercise, progressively increasing the intensity as your strength grows.

Remember to prioritize appropriate form and listen to your body to avoid injury. With regularity and determination, bodyweight exercises may convert morning workouts into excellent sessions for developing functional strength and general well-being.

Chapter 5: Balance and Stability Exercises

Incorporating balance and stability exercises into your morning training program will boost your overall fitness and establish a good tone for the rest of the day.

These exercises not only enhance physical balance and stability, but they also help with mental focus and attention. Here's a detailed guide to balance and stability exercises designed exclusively for women's early workouts:

Single-Leg Balance: Stand tall, feet hip-width apart, and shift your weight to one leg while raising the other slightly off the ground

switch sides after holding for a position for 30 seconds to one minute To make the workout more difficult, consider shutting your eyes or adding arm motions.

Stability Ball Squats: Position a stability ball between your lower back and a wall. Squat down slowly, bending your knees and supporting yourself with the ball against the wall. Aim for 10-15 repetitions while maintaining appropriate form and stability throughout.

Bosu Ball Lunges: Stand on a Bosu ball and plant one foot in the center. Step backward with the opposite foot into a lunge stance, keeping your front knee aligned with your ankle. Return to the starting position, then swap legs. To increase balance and leg strength, perform 10–12 repetitions on each leg.

Plank Variations: Incorporate side planks, plank leg lifts, and plank rotations into your workout program. These workouts work your core muscles and increase general stability. Aim for 30-60 seconds every plank variation, with emphasis on maintaining good alignment and stability.

Consider adopting Tai Chi or yoga positions that promote balance and stability, such as Tree Pose, Warrior III, or Half Moon Pose. These mind-body exercises not only help with physical balance, but also encourage relaxation and mental clarity.

Proprioceptive Training: Include activities that will test your proprioception, such as standing on a balancing board or utilizing wobble cushions. These gadgets produce an unstable surface, requiring your body to use fewer stabilizing muscles to stay balanced.

Including these balance and stability exercises in your morning workout regimen may improve your overall physical fitness, increase mental focus, and set a good tone for the day. Begin with a few exercises and progressively increase their intensity as you gain strength and stability.

Core Strengthening for Improved Stability

Women's general fitness and health benefit greatly from improving core stability and strength. These exercises not only improve stability, but they also promote good posture, reduce injury risk, and assist with daily tasks. Including these routines in your morning regimen might help you start the day with energy and vibrancy.

1. Plank Variations: Planks serve as the foundation for core strengthening. Begin with a conventional plank, keeping a straight line from head to heels and strengthening your core muscles.

To target other core muscles, go to side planks and other plank variants including forearm planks, plank twists, and plank reaches.

2. Russian Twists: Sit on the floor with your knees bent and your feet elevated, then lean back slightly and raise your feet off the ground. Twist your body from side to side while gripping a weight or medicine ball. Engage your obliques and deep core muscles.

3. Bicycle Crunches: Lie on your back, hands behind your head, and pull your knees to your chest. Extend one leg alternately while moving the opposing elbow towards the opposite knee in a cycling action, exercising both the upper and lower abdominals.

4. Dead Bug Exercise: Lie on your back, arms stretched to the ceiling, knees bent at a 90-degree angle. Lower one arm and the opposing leg to the ground, keeping your back flat, then return to the starting position and repeat on the other side.

5. *Bird Dogs:* Start on your hands and knees, then stretch one arm forward and the opposing leg backward while maintaining core engagement and hip stability. Switch sides and repeat, concentrating on balance and stability.

6. *Stability Ball Rollouts:* Kneel in front of a stability ball, lay your hands on top of it, and roll forward to stretch your body into a plank posture. Roll back to the beginning position, regulating the action with your core muscles.

Consistency is essential when including core strengthening exercises into your daily regimen. Aim for at least 10-15 minutes of focused core exercises, progressively increasing the intensity and length as your strength develops. quickly see increased stability, posture, and general strength.

Balance Exercises to Reduce the Risk of Falls

Falls are a major issue for women, particularly as they age. However, including balancing exercises in your morning routine can help lower the chance of falling and improve general stability.

Here are some extensive and detailed balancing exercises, especially designed for women:

Single-Leg Stance: Stand tall, feet hip-width apart. Lift one foot off the ground and balance on the opposite leg for 30 seconds. Switch legs and repeat. This exercise increases ankle stability and general balance.

Remember to breathe deeply and activate your core muscles throughout each exercise for best results. With dedication and patience, you willWalk in a straight line, keeping the heel of one foot squarely in front of the toes of the other with each stride. Aim for 20 steps forward and 20 steps backward. This exercise improves coordination and proprioception.

Sit on the edge of a firm chair, keeping your feet hip-width apart. Stand up without using your hands and then gently return to a sitting position.

Repeat for 10 to 15 times. Chair stands increase lower-body strength, particularly with the quadriceps and glutes, which are essential for stability.

Tree Pose: Stand with your feet hip-width apart, shift your weight to one leg, and bring the sole of the other foot to the inner thigh or calf of the standing leg. Hold hands together in front of the chest for 30 seconds. Switch sides and repeat. This yoga stance promotes balance and develops the leg muscles.

Side Leg Raises: Stand behind a chair and grab the back for support. Lift one leg directly to the side while maintaining it straight, then drop it back down. Perform 10-15 reps for each leg. Side leg lifts work the hip abductors, which are responsible for lateral stability.

Incorporate these balancing exercises into your morning routine to increase stability, lower your chance of falling, and overall quality of life.

Remember to start cautiously and progressively increase the intensity as you gain strength and confidence. Consistency is crucial to receiving the long-term advantages of these activities.

Stability Ball and Bosu Ball Workouts for Core and Balance

Starting your day with a focused workout may establish a good tone for the rest of the day. For women wishing to improve their core strength and balance, integrating stability ball and bosu ball exercises into their daily routine may be quite beneficial.

These adaptable tools work numerous muscle groups at once, improving stability, coordination, and general fitness.

Stability Ball Exercises:

Ball Crunches: Lie on the ball, supporting your lower back and keeping your feet level on the floor. Perform crunches, using your core to elevate your upper body to the sky.
Plank: Place your forearms on the ball and stretch your legs behind you while keeping a straight line from head to heels. Maintain this stance by activating your core and stabilizing muscles.

Leg Raises: Lie on your back, ball between your feet. Lift your legs to the ceiling while keeping them straight, then drop them back down without hitting the ground to target your lower abs.

Bosu Ball Exercises:

Bosu Ball Squats: Stand on the flat side of the Bosu ball, feet hip-width apart. Squat while activating your core and glutes to maintain balance.

Stand on the flat side of the Bosu ball with one leg, knee slightly bent. Maintain this position to test your balance and strengthen your core.

Push-Ups: stance your hands on the flat side of the Bosu ball and enter a plank stance. Push-ups should be performed with your core and upper body muscles engaged while stabilizing on the Bosu ball.

Benefits:

Improved Core Strength: These exercises work the core muscles, which include the abdominals, obliques, and lower back, resulting in better stability and posture.

Enhanced Balance and Coordination: The unstable surface of the stability ball and Bosu ball tests your balance, which helps to enhance coordination and proprioception.

Workouts are time-efficient since they engage numerous muscle groups at the same time.

Incorporating stability ball and Bosu ball exercises into your morning routine will help you start the day with more energy, stronger core muscles, and greater balance, putting you on track for physical and mental success.

Chapter 6: Mind-Body Connection: Yoga and Meditation

Yoga and meditation are comprehensive activities that focus on the mind-body link, improving physical, mental, and emotional health.

These ancient techniques have gained widespread appeal because of their multiple health advantages, including the capacity to relieve stress, increase flexibility, and improve general quality of life.

Yoga is a physical and mental exercise that originated in ancient India. It combines physical postures (asanas), breathing methods (pranayama), and meditation to achieve a harmonic balance of the body, mind, and spirit.

The physical postures improve flexibility, strength, and balance, while the breathing methods encourage relaxation and stress relief. Yoga also promotes mindfulness, helping practitioners to build present-moment awareness and a stronger connection with oneself.

Meditation is a technique that focuses the mind and eliminates distractions to create clarity and peace. There are different meditation approaches, such as mindfulness meditation, loving-kindness meditation, and transcendental meditation.

Meditation, regardless of style, reduces stress, anxiety, and sadness while increasing focus, creativity, and general cognitive performance.

Yoga and meditation can enhance morning exercises for women, providing several advantages. Starting the day with a yoga practice may help boost energy, enhance attention, and establish a good tone for the day. The physical postures assist to wake up the body and prepare it for the day's activities, while the breathing methods encourage relaxation and relieve morning stiffness.

Additionally, incorporating meditation into the morning practice might help women manage stress and anxiety more successfully throughout the day.

Taking a few minutes to sit quietly and focus on the breath may have a significant influence on women's mental health, leaving them feeling more focused, grounded, and resilient in the face of everyday obstacles.

Yoga and meditation are effective ways to strengthen the mind-body connection and improve general well-being. Incorporating these techniques into women's morning exercises can improve physical health, mental clarity, and emotional balance, laying the groundwork for a productive and joyful day ahead.

Gentle Yoga Poses for Flexibility and Relaxation

Gentle yoga positions are a peaceful approach to enhance flexibility and encourage relaxation, making them great for morning exercises for ladies who want to start their day with a quiet and revitalized mind-body connection. Incorporating these poses into your daily ritual will help you start the day on a good note.

Child's Pose (Balasana): Begin by kneeling on the mat, then sit back on your heels with your arms extended front, dropping your forehead to the ground. This easy stretch lengthens the spine while releasing tension in the back and shoulders.

Cat-Cow Stretch (Marjaryasana-Bitilasana): Start on your hands and knees: Inhale as you arch your back and elevate your head and tailbone (Cow Pose), then exhale as you circle your spine and tuck your chin to your chest (Cat Pose). This routine increases spinal flexibility and warms the spine.

Downward-Facing Dog (Adho Mukha Svanasana): Start in a plank posture and pull your hips up and back, producing an inverted V with your body.

Hold your hands shoulder-width apart and your feet hip-width apart. Downward Dog stretches the hamstrings, calves, and shoulders while relaxing the spine.

Seated Forward Bend (Paschimottanasana): Sit on the mat, legs outstretched in front of you. Inhale to stretch your spine, then exhale and fold forward from the hips, aiming for your feet or shins. This posture stretches the spine, hamstrings, and lower back, encouraging relaxation and serenity.

Corpse Pose (Savasana): Lie flat on your back, arms at your sides, palms up. Close your eyes and concentrate on deep, rhythmical breathing. Savasana offers for full relaxation and combines the advantages of the preceding positions.

Incorporating these mild yoga positions into a woman's morning fitness regimen may help develop flexibility, decrease tension, and build an inner serenity that will last throughout the day.

Begin with a few minutes of each posture, then gradually increase the length as your flexibility improves. Remember to listen to your body and alter postures to meet your own requirements and abilities.

Mindful Meditation Practices for Stress Reduction

Mindful meditation is an effective way to reduce stress and improve general well-being. Incorporating mindful meditation methods into your daily routine can help you develop a sense of calm, improve attention, and increase resistance to stress. Here's a complete guide to mindful meditation activities for stress reduction.

Setting the Scene: Locate a peaceful, comfortable area where you will not be interrupted. Settle into a comfortable sitting or lying posture. Close your eyes or gently look at a fixed location.

Focus on the Breath: Begin by paying attention to your breath. Consider the sensation of the breath as it enters and exits your body. Take slow, deep breaths, letting your tummy rise and fall with each inhalation and exhalation.

Body Scan: Move your focus to different regions of your body, beginning with your toes and gradually progressing up to your head. Identify any points of tension or discomfort and gradually release them with each exhale.

Mindfulness of Thought: Recognize any ideas or distractions that emerge without judgment. Simply watch them, then gently return your attention to your breath or bodily sensations.

Gratitude Practice: Take a time to think on what you are grateful for. Cultivating a grateful mindset might help to improve your outlook and lessen stress.

Visualization: Imagine yourself in a pleasant and serene setting, such as a relaxing beach or a tranquil woodland. Engage your senses by picturing the sights, sounds, and fragrances of this environment.

Mantra Meditation: As you inhale and exhale, silently repeat a relaxing mantra or phrase to yourself. Choose phrases that speak to you, such as "peace," "calm," or "I am enough."

Loving-Kindness Meditation: Extend compassion and kindness to yourself and others.

Reflection: Take a few moments to consider your meditation practice. Observe any changes in your mood, energy levels, or general sense of well-being.

Integration: Carry the advantages of your meditation practice with you all day. When you're feeling worried or overwhelmed, turn to these thoughtful strategies to discover serenity and clarity.

Incorporating mindful meditation methods into your daily routine may considerably reduce stress, increase emotional control, and improve overall well-being.

 Commit to regular practice, even if it's only for a few minutes each day, and see how it improves your overall well-being.

Breathing Techniques for Relaxation and Mental Clarity

In today's fast-paced world, finding moments of peace and mental clarity is critical for general well-being.

Incorporating breathing exercises into your everyday routine might aid in achieving this balance. Whether you're starting your day with early workouts or need a noon pick-me-up, these tactics may be used anywhere, at any time.

Deep Breathing: Start by sitting or sleeping in a comfortable posture. Close your eyes and breathe deeply through your nose, allowing your abdomen to expand completely.

Hold your breath for a few seconds, then gently exhale through your mouth to relieve any tension in your body. Repeat this cycle for a few minutes, concentrating on the rhythm of your breathing.

Counted Breaths: Counting your breaths helps you stay focused and relaxed.

Inhale deeply for four counts, then hold for four counts. exhale gently for four counts, then wait for four counts before repeating the process.
Adjust the count to your comfort level, aiming for smooth and consistent breaths.

Alternate Nostril Breathing: Sit comfortably, spine straight.Close your right nostril with your right thumb and take a deep breath in through your left.

 At the peak of your inhalation, shut your left nostril with your right ring finger while releasing your right nose, then fully exhale. Inhale via the right nostril, seal both nostrils quickly, and expel through the left nostril. Repeat this pattern for many minutes, concentrating on the flow of air and keeping a consistent beat.

Box Breathing: While breathing in this rhythm, visualize a square or box form. Inhale deeply for four counts, hold your breath for four counts, exhale for four counts, then hold your breath once more for four counts.

Repeat this cycle, focusing on the equal length of each phase and allowing your mind to become completely present in the moment.

Chapter 7: Nutrition Tips for Supporting Morning Workouts

Morning workouts may set the tone for a productive day, particularly for women who want to stay healthy and motivated.

A proper diet is essential for reaping the full advantages of these early activities. Here is some extensive and detailed dietary advice for morning workouts:

Pre-Workout Fuel: Begin your day with a balanced meal that includes carbs, proteins, and healthy fats. Choose nutritious grains such as porridge or whole wheat bread, along with lean proteins like Greek yogurt or eggs.

This combination gives long-lasting energy and promotes muscle repair.

Hydration: When you wake up, hydrate yourself to recover fluids lost while sleeping. Drink at least 8-16 ounces of water before your workout to avoid dehydration and improve performance.

Timing: Allow enough time for digestion before exercise. Aim to have a light lunch or snack with readily digested carbs and a little quantity of protein 30-60 minutes before doing exercise. This scheduling ensures that nutrients are quickly available for energy while minimizing pain during activity.

Snack Options: Choose readily digested snacks such as a banana with almond butter, a small smoothie with fruits and protein powder, or a handful of almonds and dried fruit. These solutions deliver an immediate energy boost without weighing you down.

Post-Workout Nutrition: Refuel your body within 30 minutes of your workout to aid in muscle regeneration and glycogen replenishment.

Choose a protein-packed snack, such as a protein shake, Greek yogurt with berries, or a turkey and avocado wrap on whole grain bread.

Electrolyte Balance: Include electrolyte-rich foods like bananas, coconut water, and leafy greens in your post-workout meals to replace electrolytes lost via perspiration and stay hydrated.

Listen to your body. Pay attention to how different meals make you feel before and after exercising. Experiment with several alternatives to see what works best for your body and improves your energy and performance.

Following these nutrition guidelines can help women sustain their early exercises, improve performance, and reach their fitness objectives with energy and vigor.

Pre-Workout Fueling Strategies for Energy

Strategic pre-workout feeding is critical for boosting performance during morning exercises, particularly in women. Proper eating before exercise maintains proper energy levels, improves endurance, and aids in muscle repair.

Here are some complete, detailed, and to-the-point pre-workout fueling techniques targeted for ladies who work out in the morning:

Hydration: Start your day off well by drinking plenty of water. Aim for at least 16-20 ounces of water when you get up to restore fluids lost while sleeping and kickstart your metabolism. Adequate water boosts energy levels and avoids dehydration during exercise.

Carbohydrates: Eat readily digested carbs 30-60 minutes before exercise. Choose fruit (banana, apple), full grain bread, or oats. Carbohydrates give easily accessible energy to power exercises and regulate blood sugar levels.

Protein: Combine carbs and a modest quantity of protein to improve muscle repair and recovery. Greek yogurt, a hard-boiled egg, and a protein drink are some examples. To avoid pain when exercising, use an easily digested protein source.

Fats: While fats take longer to digest, eating a little quantity of healthy fats can give long-lasting energy during the workout. Consider spreading a dollop of nut butter on toast or putting avocado into a smoothie.

Timing: Allow ample time to digest before beginning the workout. Eat 30-60 minutes before exercise to avoid pain and enhance nutrition absorption.

To see what works best for you experiment with time

Consider taking caffeine or BCAAs (branched-chain amino acids) supplements to enhance your energy and assist your muscles. However, be aware of individual sensitivities and contact with a healthcare practitioner before incorporating supplements into your regimen.

Listen to your body. Pay attention to how various diets influence your energy and performance. Everyone's dietary requirements and tolerances differ, so modify your pre-workout fuelling approach based on how your body reacts.

Women who follow these pre-workout nutrition tactics designed for morning exercises can boost their energy levels, increase their performance, and improve their overall fitness results. Remember to prioritize consistency and pay attention to your body's messages in order to attain your fitness objectives successfully.

Post-Workout Nutrition for Recovery and Muscle Repair

Post-workout nourishment is essential for women who work out in the morning to help with recovery and muscle restoration.

A nutritious post-workout breakfast or snack should include protein, carbs, and water to replace glycogen reserves, repair muscle tissue, and hydrate the body.

Protein is necessary for muscle repair and development. Women should have around 20–30 grams of high-quality protein within 30 minutes to an hour of their morning activity.

Eggs, Greek yogurt, tofu, and protein shakes prepared with whey or plant-based protein powder are all good sources of protein.

Carbohydrates help to replace glycogen reserves, which are lost during activity. Choosing complex carbs such as whole grains, fruits, and vegetables promotes a consistent flow of energy and aids in muscle repair. Aim for 30-50 grams of carbs after the workout.

In addition to protein and carbs, water is essential for proper recovery. Women should drink lots of water before, during, and after their workouts to replenish fluids lost via perspiration. Coconut water or sports drinks can also help replace electrolytes lost during exercise.

Some women may benefit from incorporating a little quantity of healthy fats into their post-workout meal to promote joint health and hormone production. Avocado, almonds, or seeds can be added to a post-workout smoothie or salad to give necessary fats.

Timing is also critical for post-workout nourishment. Consuming a healthy breakfast or snack 30 minutes to an hour after exercise can help the body recover and repair muscular tissue.

To assist recovery and muscle regeneration, women who exercise in the morning should consume a well-balanced post-workout meal or snack that includes protein, carbs, water, and potentially some healthy fats.

Women may improve their performance and achieve their fitness objectives by fuelling their bodies with the appropriate nutrition at the right time.

Hydration and Electrolyte Balance for Optimal Performance

To improve their performance and general health, women who exercise in the morning must maintain sufficient hydration and electrolyte balance.

Hydration is required to sustain basic functioning, regulate body temperature, and deliver nutrients to cells. Electrolytes are essential for muscular contraction, neuron function, and fluid equilibrium.

Women must start the day with appropriate fluids before beginning their workout. To start your day off right, drink at least 16–20 ounces of water.

Throughout the morning, sip water to stay hydrated. Adding a slice of lemon or a sprinkle of salt to your drink will help replace electrolytes lost while sleeping.

Women should consume water throughout their workout, especially if it is vigorous or lengthy. Drink water often, aiming for 7-10 ounces every 10-20 minutes while exercising.

For workouts lasting more than an hour or in hot weather, try drinking a sports drink containing electrolytes to restore those lost via sweating.

After the workout, concentrate on drinking and replacing electrolytes. Drink water or an electrolyte-containing recovery drink within 30 minutes after finishing your workout to help with recovery and muscle restoration. Adding protein, such as a protein shake or a small snack, can help with muscle rehabilitation.

In addition to hydration, women should monitor their electrolyte balance. A balanced diet high in fruits, vegetables, whole grains, and lean meats delivers the necessary electrolytes.

Consuming foods such as bananas, spinach, yogurt, and almonds can help replace potassium, calcium, and magnesium stores.

For women to function well during early exercise, appropriate hydration and electrolyte balance are critical. Start the day with proper hydration, refill fluids while active, and concentrate on rehydration and electrolyte restoration afterward.

Maintain a well-balanced diet to support your electrolyte levels and general health.

Chapter 8: Creating a Sustainable Morning Workout Routine

Establishing a consistent morning fitness program benefits not just physical health but also mental well-being and general productivity throughout the day.

For women, including morning exercises in their daily schedule can be especially beneficial since it sets a good tone for the day and gives them concentrated time for self-care. Here's how to develop a complete and sustained morning workout routine:

Set realistic objectives: Start by establishing attainable fitness objectives based on your specific needs and fitness level. Setting clear, quantifiable, and reasonable objectives, whether they be for cardiovascular health, strength, or flexibility, can help you stay motivated and measure your progress.

Choose Enjoyable Activities: Choose workouts and activities that you actually love. Whether it's yoga, running, swimming, or dancing, including things you enjoy into your daily routine can help you stick to it in the long run.

Start Slowly: If you're new to morning exercises, begin with shorter sessions and gradually increase the time and intensity as your fitness improves. This strategy will assist to minimize burnout and lower the chance of harm.

Schedule Regular Workouts: Consistency is essential for developing a sustainable morning training regimen. Set certain days and times for your workouts and treat them like non-negotiable meetings with yourself.

Prioritize recuperation: Allow yourself adequate rest and recuperation between sessions to avoid overtraining and injury. Stretching, foam rolling, and restorative yoga may all help you recuperate and relax your muscles.

Fuel Your Body: Before or after your morning workout, eat a nutritious meal to provide your body the energy it needs to perform well and recuperate. Choose nutrient-dense meals that include carbs, protein, and healthy fats.

Stay Hydrated: Drink lots of water before, during, and after your workout to keep your body hydrated and functioning properly. Proper hydration is vital for peak performance and wellbeing.

Listen to your body. Pay attention to how your body feels throughout exercise and modify accordingly. If you're tired or in pain, it's best to rest and recuperate instead than pushing through possibly hazardous discomfort.

By following these steps and being committed to your morning fitness program, you may establish a long-term practice that benefits your physical and emotional health as a woman.

 Remember to be patient with yourself and recognize your accomplishments along the road.

Setting Realistic Goals and Tracking Progress

Setting realistic objectives and measuring progress are critical components of any successful fitness journey, particularly early exercise for women.

By setting attainable goals and tracking your progress, you may stay motivated, be consistent, and finally accomplish your intended outcomes.

To begin, develop SMART goals that are specific, measurable, achievable, relevant, and time-bound. For example, instead of just wanting to "get fit," a more particular goal may be to "complete a 30-minute morning workout three times a week for the next three months."

This objective is explicit in terms of duration and frequency, quantifiable in terms of time spent exercising, attainable for most people with a consistent routine, relevant to improving fitness levels, and time-bound with a three-month timeline.

Once you've set your goals, tracking your progress is critical to ensuring you're on target. This may be done in a variety of ways, including maintaining an exercise log, utilizing fitness monitoring apps, or simply recording completed workouts on a calendar.

Tracking progress helps you to assess how far you've come, spot patterns or trends, and make changes to your routine.

Women who incorporate morning workouts into their routines benefit from greater energy levels throughout the day, improved mood and mental clarity, and enhanced metabolism. To avoid fatigue or damage, start gently and listen to your body. Begin with shorter exercises, then progressively increase the intensity and length as your strength and endurance improve.

Morning workouts need a high level of consistency. Establishing and sticking to a regular regimen can help turn exercise into a habit rather than a hassle. Setting modest milestones along the road might create a sense of accomplishment and incentive to continue.

Setting reasonable objectives and evaluating progress are critical components of effective morning exercises for women. By setting clear, quantifiable goals and tracking your progress, you may stay motivated, consistent, and eventually achieve your fitness goals.

Incorporating Variety and Adaptability for Long-Term Success

Starting the day with a morning workout sets a good tone for the remainder of the day, especially for women who want to prioritize their health and fitness.

Incorporating variation and adaptation into morning exercises is critical for long-term success, ensuring that women not only meet but also maintain their fitness objectives.

Variety is essential for keeping early exercises exciting and successful. Women can use several forms of activities, such as aerobics, weight training, yoga, or Pilates, to target different muscle areas and avoid boredom.

Cardio workouts such as running, cycling, and jumping rope enhance heart health and stamina, and strength training with body weight or free weights increases muscle mass and metabolism. Yoga and Pilates promote flexibility, balance, and stress alleviation, therefore improving general well-being.

Furthermore, for long-term success, morning workouts must be tailored to individual preferences and schedules. Some women choose high-intensity interval training (HIIT) for a rapid but intense workout, while others prefer a longer, more leisurely session.

Including outdoor activities such as jogging or hiking may offer diversity and excitement to morning exercises, allowing women to reconnect with nature while exercising.

Incorporating variation and adaptation into morning exercises entails listening to your body and altering the intensity or time as necessary. Women should pay attention to how their bodies feel each day and adjust their training routine accordingly.

This might entail taking rest days, performing active recovery with light workouts like walking or stretching, or modifying the intensity based on energy levels and recovery progress.

Women's early exercises require consistency to be successful over time. Women who include diversity and adaptability into their routines can stay motivated, avoid plateaus, and continue their fitness journey for years to come.

Whether it's attempting new exercises, modifying workout lengths, or listening to their bodies, embracing diversity and adaptation ensures that morning workouts stay pleasurable and beneficial for women looking to improve their long-term health and fitness.

Troubleshooting Common Barriers and Adjusting the Routine

Morning exercises can help women start their day with energy and vibrancy. However, numerous frequent impediments might impede consistency and efficacy.

Understanding these hurdles and changing your training regimen properly will help you overcome challenges and reach your fitness objectives.

Common barriers:

Lack of Time: Women frequently juggle many duties, leaving little time for exercise.

Low Energy Levels: Lack of sleep or a sluggish metabolism can make mornings difficult.

Lack of Motivation: Early mornings can be demotivating, particularly during the winter months.

Physical Discomfort: Previous workouts that left muscles stiff or with joint ache might inhibit morning activity.

Environmental Factors: Dark mornings, chilly weather, and loud surroundings may discourage outside activity.

Changing the Routine

Set Realistic Goals: Create brief, doable exercises that are targeted to your available time and energy levels.

Prioritize Sleep: Create a consistent nighttime routine to ensure you get enough sleep.

Dynamic Warm-ups: Use dynamic stretches and brief exercise to wake up your muscles and improve circulation.
To enhance motivation, listen to inspiring music, read encouraging quotations, or work out with friends.

Adapt to Comfort: Choose indoor exercises or purchase weather-appropriate outdoor gear.

Gradual Progress: Begin with moderate workouts and gradually raise the intensity to avoid overexertion.

Flexible Schedule: Allow for flexibility in workout scheduling to allow unforeseen interruptions.

Mindful Nutrition: Before exercising, fuel your body with a light, balanced breakfast or snack to improve performance.

Post-Workout repair: Use cooldown stretches and stay hydrated to improve muscle repair.
Positive reinforcement involves celebrating little triumphs and acknowledging progress in order to maintain motivation.

Women may overcome obstacles and gain the many advantages of regular exercise by changing their morning workout regimen and addressing typical roadblocks. Consistency, adaptation, and self-care are essential for accomplishing long-term fitness goals and leading a healthy lifestyle.

CONCLUSION

Morning exercises for women have several physical, mental, and emotional benefits that contribute to overall health and a higher quality of life.

This extensive investigation demonstrates that exercising in the morning hours has considerable benefits for women in a variety of facets of their lives.

Morning workouts promote greater metabolism, cardiovascular health, and weight control. The metabolic surge experienced during exercise sets a good tone for the remainder of the day, encouraging increased calorie expenditure and fat utilization.

Regular morning exercise routines have been shown to lower rates of chronic illnesses such as diabetes, hypertension, and obesity, improving lifespan and optimal health outcomes.

The psychological benefits of early exercise for women cannot be overemphasized.

Exercise releases endorphins, which function as a natural mood booster, lowering stress, anxiety, and depression symptoms.

This boost in mood and mental clarity leads to increased productivity, attention, and resilience throughout the day.

The sense of satisfaction gained from finishing a morning workout sets a good tone for the rest of the day, encouraging an attitude of achievement and self-efficacy.

Morning workouts are a powerful tool for women, allowing them to prioritize their physical and mental health despite the pressures of everyday life. Women can build a regular habit that corresponds with their objectives and beliefs by setting aside specific morning exercise times.

This proactive attitude to self-care not only fosters a sense of self-worth and empowerment, but it also sets a strong example for others, encouraging friends, family, and communities to prioritize their health and well-being.

In essence, morning exercises provide women with a comprehensive approach to health and vitality, including physical, mental, and emotional well-being.
Women who embrace the benefits of early morning exercise can go on a road to improved health, happiness, and fulfillment in all parts of their lives.

THANK YOU PAGE

Thank you for selecting this book. Your support is really appreciated. Similarly, I am grateful for the purchase of this book.

Your input is valuable; please share your ideas in a review. It serves as a reference for future improvements. Enjoy reading and utilizing it!

Workout planner for tracking progress over time

Weekly
Workout Planner

Week : _______________

Month: _______________

Sunday

Monday

Tuesday

Goals

Goals

Goals

Wednesday

Thursday

Friday

Goals

Goals

Goals

Saturday

Water Tracker

Goals

Mood

Motivation ___________________________
____
____
____
____
____

Weekly
Workout Planner

Week : _______________

Month: _______________

Sunday	Monday	Tuesday
Goals	Goals	Goals

Wednesday	Thursday	Friday
Goals	Goals	Goals

Saturday

Water Tracker

Goals

Mood

Motivation _______________________________________
____
____
____
____

Weekly
Workout Planner

Week : _______________

Month: _______________

Sunday

Monday

Tuesday

Goals

Goals

Goals

Wednesday

Thursday

Friday

Goals

Goals

Goals

Saturday

Water Tracker

Goals

Mood

Motivation ________________________________

____

____

____

____

Weekly
Workout Planner

Week :_______________

Month:_______________

Sunday   Monday   Tuesday

Goals   Goals   Goals

Wednesday   Thursday   Friday

Goals   Goals   Goals

Saturday   Water Tracker

Goals   **Mood**

Motivation _______________________________

____

____

____

Weekly
Workout Planner

Week :_______________

Month: _______________

Sunday

Goals

Monday

Goals

Tuesday

Goals

Wednesday

Goals

Thursday

Goals

Friday

Goals

Saturday

Goals

Water Tracker

Mood

Goals

Motivation ____

____

____

____

____

Weekly
Workout Planner

Week : ___________________

Month: ___________________

Sunday

Monday

Tuesday

Goals

Goals

Goals

Wednesday

Thursday

Friday

Goals

Goals

Goals

Saturday

Water Tracker

Goals

Mood

Motivation ____

Weekly
Workout Planner

Week :_______________

Month:_______________

Sunday	Monday	Tuesday
Goals	Goals	Goals

Wednesday	Thursday	Friday
Goals	Goals	Goals

Saturday

Water Tracker

Goals

Mood

Motivation

Weekly
Workout Planner

Week : _______________

Month: _______________

Sunday	Monday	Tuesday
Goals	Goals	Goals

Wednesday	Thursday	Friday
Goals	Goals	Goals

Saturday

Water Tracker

Goals

Mood

Motivation _________________________________

Weekly
Workout Planner

Week :_______________

Month:_______________

Sunday   Monday   Tuesday

Goals   Goals   **Goals**

Wednesday   Thursday   Friday

Goals   **Goals**   Goals

Saturday   Water Tracker

Goals   **Mood**

Motivation ________________________________

Weekly
Workout Planner

Week : _______________

Month: _______________

Sunday

Monday

Tuesday

Goals

Goals

Goals

Wednesday

Thursday

Friday

Goals

Goals

Goals

Saturday

Water Tracker

Goals

Mood

Motivation ______________________________

____

____

____

____

Weekly
Workout Planner

Week :_______________

Month:_______________

Sunday	Monday	Tuesday
Goals	Goals	**Goals**

Wednesday	Thursday	Friday
Goals	**Goals**	Goals

Saturday	Water Tracker
Goals	**Mood**

Motivation ______________________________
____
____
____
____

Weekly
Workout Planner

Week :_______________

Month: _______________

Sunday

Monday

Tuesday

Goals

Goals

Goals

Wednesday

Thursday

Friday

Goals

Goals

Goals

Saturday

Water Tracker

Goals

Mood

Motivation ________________________

Weekly
Workout Planner

Week :_______________

Month:_______________

Sunday

Monday

Tuesday

Goals

Goals

Goals

Wednesday

Thursday

Friday

Goals

Goals

Goals

Saturday

Water Tracker

Goals

Mood

Motivation _______________

Weekly
Workout Planner

Week : __________________

Month: __________________

Sunday	Monday	Tuesday
Goals	Goals	Goals

Wednesday	Thursday	Friday
Goals	Goals	Goals

Saturday

Water Tracker

Goals

Mood

Motivation ________________________________
____
____
____
____

Weekly
Workout Planner

Week :_______________

Month:_______________

Sunday	Monday	Tuesday
Goals	Goals	**Goals**

Wednesday	Thursday	Friday
Goals	**Goals**	Goals

Saturday   Water Tracker

Goals   **Mood**

Motivation _______________________________

____

____

____

____

Weekly
Workout Planner

Week :_______________

Month:_______________

Sunday	Monday	Tuesday
Goals	Goals	Goals

Wednesday	Thursday	Friday
Goals	Goals	Goals

Saturday

Water Tracker

Goals

Mood

Motivation _________________________________

Weekly
Workout Planner

Week :_______________

Month: _______________

Sunday   Monday   Tuesday

Goals   Goals   **Goals**

Wednesday   Thursday   Friday

Goals   **Goals**   Goals

Saturday   Water Tracker

Goals   **Mood**

Motivation _______________________________
____
____
____
____

Weekly
Workout Planner

Week :_______________

Month: _______________

Sunday

Monday

Tuesday

Goals

Goals

Goals

Wednesday

Thursday

Friday

Goals

Goals

Goals

Saturday

Water Tracker

Goals

Mood

Motivation ________________________

Weekly
Workout Planner

Week :________________

Month:________________

Sunday

Monday

Tuesday

Goals

Goals

Goals

Wednesday

Thursday

Friday

Goals

Goals

Goals

Saturday

Water Tracker

Goals

Mood

Motivation ____

____

____

____

____

Weekly
Workout Planner

Week :________________

Month:________________

Sunday   Monday   Tuesday

Goals   Goals   Goals

Wednesday   Thursday   Friday

Goals   Goals   Goals

Saturday   Water Tracker

Goals

Mood

Motivation ________________________________

Weekly
Workout Planner

Week : _______________

Month: _______________

Sunday	Monday	Tuesday
Goals	Goals	**Goals**

Wednesday	Thursday	Friday
Goals	**Goals**	Goals

Saturday	Water Tracker
Goals	**Mood**

Mood

Motivation ___________________________

____
____
____
____

Weekly
Workout Planner

Week :_________________

Month:_______________

Sunday

Monday

Tuesday

Goals

Goals

Goals

Wednesday

Thursday

Friday

Goals

Goals

Goals

Saturday

Water Tracker

Goals

Mood

Motivation ________________________________

Weekly
Workout Planner

Week :______________

Month:______________

Sunday	Monday	Tuesday
Goals	Goals	**Goals**

Wednesday	Thursday	Friday
Goals	**Goals**	Goals

Saturday	Water Tracker
Goals	**Mood**

Motivation ____
____
____
____
____

Weekly
Workout Planner

Week : ________________

Month: ________________

Sunday

Monday

Tuesday

Goals

Goals

Goals

Wednesday

Thursday

Friday

Goals

Goals

Goals

Saturday

Water Tracker

Goals

Mood

Motivation

Weekly
Workout Planner

Week: ___________

Month: ___________

Sunday	Monday	Tuesday
Goals	Goals	Goals

Wednesday	Thursday	Friday
Goals	Goals	Goals

Saturday

Goals

Water Tracker

Mood

Motivation ___________________________

____

____

____

____

Weekly
Workout Planner

Week : _______________

Month: _______________

Sunday

Monday

Tuesday

Goals

Goals

Goals

Wednesday

Thursday

Friday

Goals

Goals

Goals

Saturday

Water Tracker

Goals

Mood

Motivation _______________________________

Weekly
Workout Planner

Week : ___________

Month: ___________

Sunday	Monday	Tuesday
Goals	Goals	Goals

Wednesday	Thursday	Friday
Goals	Goals	Goals

Saturday	Water Tracker
Goals	**Mood**

Motivation ____________________

____

____

____

____

Weekly
Workout Planner

Week : _______________

Month: _______________

Sunday	Monday	Tuesday
Goals	Goals	**Goals**

Wednesday	Thursday	Friday
Goals	**Goals**	Goals

Saturday

Water Tracker

Goals

Mood

Motivation _______________

Weekly
Workout Planner

Week :_______________

Month: _______________

Sunday   Monday   Tuesday

Goals   Goals   **Goals**

Wednesday   Thursday   Friday

Goals   **Goals**   Goals

Saturday   Water Tracker

Goals   **Mood**

Motivation _____________________________

____

____

____

____

Weekly
Workout Planner

Week :________________

Month: ________________

Sunday

Monday

Tuesday

Goals

Goals

Goals

Wednesday

Thursday

Friday

Goals

Goals

Goals

Saturday

Water Tracker

Goals

Mood

Motivation

Weekly
Workout Planner

Week : _______________

Month: _______________

Sunday	Monday	Tuesday
Goals	Goals	**Goals**

Wednesday	Thursday	Friday
Goals	**Goals**	Goals

Saturday

Water Tracker

Goals

Mood

Motivation _______________________________

Weekly
Workout Planner

Week :______________

Month:______________

Sunday

Goals

Monday

Goals

Tuesday

Goals

Wednesday

Goals

Thursday

Goals

Friday

Goals

Saturday

Goals

Water Tracker

Mood

Motivation ________________________________
____
____
____
____

Weekly
Workout Planner

Week : _______________

Month: _______________

Sunday   Monday   Tuesday

Goals   Goals   Goals

Wednesday   Thursday   Friday

Goals   Goals   Goals

Saturday   Water Tracker

Goals   **Mood**

Motivation _______________________________

Weekly
Workout Planner

Week : _______________

Month: _______________

Sunday

Monday

Tuesday

Goals

Goals

Goals

Wednesday

Thursday

Friday

Goals

Goals

Goals

Saturday

Water Tracker

Goals

Mood

Motivation _______________________________________

____

____

____

____

Weekly
Workout Planner

Week :_______________

Month:_______________

Sunday	Monday	Tuesday
Goals	Goals	**Goals**

Wednesday	Thursday	Friday
Goals	**Goals**	Goals

Saturday	Water Tracker
Goals	**Mood**

Motivation ________________________

____

____

____

____

Weekly
Workout Planner

Week : _______________

Month: _______________

Sunday	Monday	Tuesday
Goals	Goals	Goals

Wednesday	Thursday	Friday
Goals	Goals	Goals

Saturday

Goals

Water Tracker

Mood

Motivation _________________________
____
____
____
____

Weekly
Workout Planner

Week : _______________

Month: _______________

Sunday   Monday   Tuesday

Goals   Goals   **Goals**

Wednesday   Thursday   Friday

Goals   **Goals**   Goals

Saturday   Water Tracker

Goals   **Mood**

Motivation _________________________

Weekly

Workout Planner

Week :_______________

Month:_______________

Sunday	Monday	Tuesday
Goals	Goals	Goals

Wednesday	Thursday	Friday
Goals	Goals	Goals

Saturday

Water Tracker

Goals

Mood

Motivation _______________

Weekly
Workout Planner

Week : _______________

Month: _______________

Sunday

Monday

Tuesday

Goals

Goals

Goals

Wednesday

Thursday

Friday

Goals

Goals

Goals

Saturday

Water Tracker

Goals

Mood

Motivation _______________________________

____

____

____

____

Weekly
Workout Planner

Week : _______________

Month: _______________

Sunday	Monday	Tuesday
Goals	Goals	Goals

Wednesday	Thursday	Friday
Goals	Goals	Goals

Saturday

Water Tracker

Goals

Mood

😖 😁 😐 🙂 🙁

Motivation ______________________
____
____
____
____

Weekly
Workout Planner

Week : _______________

Month: _______________

Sunday

Monday

Tuesday

Goals

Goals

Goals

Wednesday

Thursday

Friday

Goals

Goals

Goals

Saturday

Water Tracker

Goals

Mood

Motivation _______________________________
____
____
____
____

Weekly
Workout Planner

Week :__________________

Month:__________________

Sunday

Monday

Tuesday

Goals

Goals

Goals

Wednesday

Thursday

Friday

Goals

Goals

Goals

Saturday

Water Tracker

Goals

Mood

Motivation _______________________

Weekly
Workout Planner

Week: _______________

Month: _______________

Sunday

Goals

Monday

Goals

Tuesday

Goals

Wednesday

Goals

Thursday

Goals

Friday

Goals

Saturday

Goals

Water Tracker

Mood

Motivation

____
____
____
____
____

Weekly
Workout Planner

Week: ___________

Month: ___________

Sunday

Monday

Tuesday

Goals

Goals

Goals

Wednesday

Thursday

Friday

Goals

Goals

Goals

Saturday

Water Tracker

Goals

Mood

Motivation ________________________

Weekly
Workout Planner

Week : _______________

Month: _______________

Sunday	Monday	Tuesday
Goals	Goals	**Goals**

Wednesday	Thursday	Friday
Goals	**Goals**	Goals

Saturday

Water Tracker

Goals

Mood

Motivation _______________________________
____
____
____
____

Weekly
Workout Planner

Week :_______________

Month:_______________

Sunday

Monday

Tuesday

Goals

Goals

Goals

Wednesday

Thursday

Friday

Goals

Goals

Goals

Saturday

Water Tracker

Goals

Mood

Motivation _______________

Weekly
Workout Planner

Week :________________

Month: ________________

Sunday

Monday

Tuesday

Goals

Goals

Goals

Wednesday

Thursday

Friday

Goals

Goals

Goals

Saturday

Water Tracker

Goals

Mood

Motivation ________________________________

Weekly
Workout Planner

Week :_______________

Month: _______________

Sunday   Monday   Tuesday

Goals   Goals   Goals

Wednesday   Thursday   Friday

Goals   Goals   Goals

Saturday   Water Tracker

Goals

Mood

Motivation ___________________________

Weekly
Workout Planner

Week :______________

Month:______________

Sunday

Monday

Tuesday

Goals

Goals

Goals

Wednesday

Thursday

Friday

Goals

Goals

Goals

Saturday

Water Tracker

Goals

Mood

Motivation ____
____
____
____
____

Weekly
Workout Planner

Week :______________

Month: ______________

Sunday

Monday

Tuesday

Goals

Goals

Goals

Wednesday

Thursday

Friday

Goals

Goals

Goals

Saturday

Water Tracker

Goals

Mood

Motivation ________________________________

Weekly
Workout Planner

Week :_________________

Month: _______________

Sunday   Monday   Tuesday

Goals   Goals   Goals

Wednesday   Thursday   Friday

Goals   Goals   Goals

Saturday   Water Tracker

Goals   Mood

Motivation

Weekly
Workout Planner

Week : _______________

Month: _______________

Sunday	Monday	Tuesday
Goals	Goals	Goals

Wednesday	Thursday	Friday
Goals	Goals	Goals

Saturday

Goals

Water Tracker

Mood

Motivation ________________________________

____

____

____

____

Weekly
Workout Planner

Week :_______________

Month:_______________

Sunday	Monday	Tuesday
Goals	Goals	**Goals**

Wednesday	Thursday	Friday
Goals	**Goals**	Goals

Saturday	Water Tracker
Goals	**Mood**

Mood

Motivation ___________________________________
____
____
____
____

Weekly
Workout Planner

Week :_______________

Month: _______________

Sunday

Monday

Tuesday

Goals

Goals

Goals

Wednesday

Thursday

Friday

Goals

Goals

Goals

Saturday

Water Tracker

Goals

Mood

Motivation __________________

Weekly
Workout Planner

Week : _______________

Month: _______________

Sunday

Monday

Tuesday

Goals

Goals

Goals

Wednesday

Thursday

Friday

Goals

Goals

Goals

Saturday

Water Tracker

Goals

Mood

Motivation

Weekly
Workout Planner

Week : _______________

Month: _______________

Sunday

Monday

Tuesday

Goals

Goals

Goals

Wednesday

Thursday

Friday

Goals

Goals

Goals

Saturday

Water Tracker

Goals

Mood

Motivation _______________________________
____
____
____
____

Weekly
Workout Planner

Week :________________

Month:________________

Sunday	Monday	Tuesday
Goals	Goals	**Goals**

Wednesday	Thursday	Friday
Goals	**Goals**	Goals

Saturday	Water Tracker
Goals	**Mood**

Motivation _______________________
____
____
____
____

Weekly
Workout Planner

Week : _______________

Month: _______________

Sunday

Monday

Tuesday

Goals

Goals

Goals

Wednesday

Thursday

Friday

Goals

Goals

Goals

Saturday

Water Tracker

Goals

Mood

Motivation _______________________________

Weekly
Workout Planner

Week :_______________

Month:_______________

Sunday	Monday	Tuesday
Goals	Goals	Goals

Wednesday	Thursday	Friday
Goals	Goals	Goals

Saturday

Water Tracker

Goals

Mood

Motivation _______________

Weekly
Workout Planner

Week :________________

Month: ________________

Sunday	Monday	Tuesday
Goals	Goals	Goals

Wednesday	Thursday	Friday
Goals	Goals	Goals

Saturday

Water Tracker

Goals

Mood

Motivation _______________________

Weekly
Workout Planner

Week: _______________

Month: _______________

Sunday	Monday	Tuesday
Goals	Goals	**Goals**

Wednesday	Thursday	Friday
Goals	**Goals**	Goals

Saturday	Water Tracker
Goals	**Mood**

Motivation ____

____

____

____

____

Weekly
Workout Planner

Week : _______________

Month: _______________

Sunday	Monday	Tuesday
Goals	Goals	Goals

Wednesday	Thursday	Friday
Goals	Goals	Goals

Saturday	Water Tracker
Goals	**Mood**

Motivation _______________________________

____

____

____

____

Weekly
Workout Planner

Week :_______________

Month:_______________

Sunday	Monday	Tuesday
Goals	Goals	Goals

Wednesday	Thursday	Friday
Goals	Goals	Goals

Saturday

Water Tracker

Goals

Mood

Motivation _______________

Weekly
Workout Planner

Week : _______________

Month: _______________

Sunday	Monday	Tuesday
Goals	Goals	**Goals**

Wednesday	Thursday	Friday
Goals	**Goals**	Goals

Saturday

Water Tracker

Goals

Mood

Motivation _______________________________________
____
____
____
____

Weekly
Workout Planner

Week : _______________

Month: _______________

Sunday	Monday	Tuesday
Goals	Goals	**Goals**

Wednesday	Thursday	Friday
Goals	**Goals**	Goals

Saturday

Goals

Water Tracker

Mood

Motivation _______________________________

Weekly
Workout Planner

Week : _______________

Month: _______________

Sunday	Monday	Tuesday
Goals	Goals	Goals

Wednesday	Thursday	Friday
Goals	Goals	Goals

Saturday

Water Tracker

Goals

Mood

Motivation

Weekly
Workout Planner

Week : _______________

Month: _______________

Sunday

Goals

Monday

Goals

Tuesday

Goals

Wednesday

Thursday

Friday

Goals

Goals

Goals

Saturday

Water Tracker

Goals

Mood

Motivation ___________________________________

Weekly
Workout Planner

Week : _______________

Month: _______________

Sunday

Goals

Monday

Goals

Tuesday

Goals

Wednesday

Goals

Thursday

Goals

Friday

Goals

Saturday

Goals

Water Tracker

Mood

Motivation _______________

Weekly
Workout Planner

Week : _______________

Month: _______________

Sunday	Monday	Tuesday
Goals	Goals	**Goals**

Wednesday	Thursday	Friday
Goals	**Goals**	Goals

Saturday

Water Tracker

Goals

Mood

Motivation _________________________________
____
____
____
____

Weekly
Workout Planner

Week : ___________________

Month: ___________________

Sunday

Monday

Tuesday

Goals

Goals

Goals

Wednesday

Thursday

Friday

Goals

Goals

Goals

Saturday

Water Tracker

Goals

Mood

Motivation _____________________________
____
____
____
____

Weekly
Workout Planner

Week : _______________

Month: _______________

Sunday

Monday

Tuesday

Goals

Goals

Goals

Wednesday

Thursday

Friday

Goals

Goals

Goals

Saturday

Water Tracker

Goals

Mood

Motivation _______________________________

____

____

____

____

Weekly
Workout Planner

Week :______________

Month: ______________

Sunday

Monday

Tuesday

Goals

Goals

Goals

Wednesday

Thursday

Friday

Goals

Goals

Goals

Saturday

Water Tracker

Goals

Mood

Motivation

Weekly
Workout Planner

Week : _______________

Month: _______________

Sunday

Monday

Tuesday

Goals

Goals

Goals

Wednesday

Thursday

Friday

Goals

Goals

Goals

Saturday

Water Tracker

Goals

Mood

Motivation ____________________________

Weekly
Workout Planner

Week : _______________

Month: _______________

Sunday

Monday

Tuesday

Goals

Goals

Goals

Wednesday

Thursday

Friday

Goals

Goals

Goals

Saturday

Water Tracker

Goals

Mood

Motivation _______________________________

____

____

____

____

Weekly
Workout Planner

Week :_______________

Month:_______________

Sunday	Monday	Tuesday
Goals	Goals	**Goals**

Wednesday	Thursday	Friday
Goals	**Goals**	Goals

Saturday	Water Tracker
Goals	**Mood**

Motivation _______________
____
____
____
____

Weekly
Workout Planner

Week : _______________

Month: _______________

Sunday

Goals

Monday

Goals

Tuesday

Goals

Wednesday

Goals

Thursday

Goals

Friday

Goals

Saturday

Goals

Water Tracker

Mood

Motivation

____
____
____
____
____

Weekly
Workout Planner

Week :_______________

Month:_____________

Sunday

Monday

Tuesday

Goals

Goals

Goals

Wednesday

Thursday

Friday

Goals

Goals

Goals

Saturday

Water Tracker

Goals

Mood

Motivation ____

Weekly
Workout Planner

Week : _______________

Month: _______________

Sunday

Monday

Tuesday

Goals

Goals

Goals

Wednesday

Thursday

Friday

Goals

Goals

Goals

Saturday

Water Tracker

Goals

Mood

Motivation _______________